Vitamin-Mineral Supplements

CW01091365

THE DOCTORS' PLAN FOR

Vitamin-Mineral Supplements

•

ELIZABETH SOMER, MA, RD
AND THE HEALTH MEDIA
EDITORIAL PANEL

foulsham

LONDON • NEW YORK • TORONTO • SYDNEY

foulsham
Yeovil Road, Slough, Berkshire SL1 4JH

ISBN 0–572–01798–7

Printed in Great Britain by
St Edmundsbury Press Ltd, Bury St Edmunds, Suffolk

Contents

1
A Realistic View Of Vitamin-Mineral Supplements

Evidence linking diet with heart disease, cancer, diabetes, and high blood pressure has made people aware of the need to take charge of their health and nutrition. Individuals not only want to avoid crippling diseases, they want to feel their best and maintain their vitality.

Nutrition is a new science. Many of the vitamins were discovered within the last few decades and the functions, interactions, and storage of these essential nutrients within the body are not completely understood.

No other topic in nutrition has stimulated more debate than has vitamin-mineral supplements in the diet.

The RDAs: Guidelines Not Gospel

The Recommended Daily Allowances (RDAs) are suggested levels of essential

Table 1 Recommended Daily Allowances*

Protein	10% of energy requirement
Vitamin A	750 μg
Vitamin B_1 (thiamin)	0.4 mg per 1000 kcal.
Vitamin B_2 (riboflavin)	
Men	1.6 mg
Women	1.3 mg
Vitamin B_3 (niacin)	
Men	18 mg
Women	15 mg
Vitamin B_6 (US RDA)	
Men	2.2 mg
Women	2.0 mg
Vitamin B_{12} (US RDA)	3.0 μg
Vitamin C (ascorbic acid)	30 mg
Vitamin D	
Children	7.5 μg
Pregnant and breastfeeding women	10 μg
Adults not exposed to sunlight	10 μg
Folic acid (folacin)	
Adults (US RDA)	400 μg
Pregnant women	800 μg
Calcium	500 mg
Pregnant and breast-feeding women and children have a higher requirement.	
Iodine (US RDA)	150 μg
Iron	
Men	10 mg
Women	12 mg
Pregnant and breastfeeding women	13–15 mg
Magnesium (US RDA)	
Adults	350 mg
Pregnant, breastfeeding and menstruating women	450 mg
Phosphorus (US RDA)	800 mg

*UK adult unless otherwise stated

nutrients considered adequate to meet the nutritional needs of healthy individuals. (*Table 1, Page 8*) These guidelines have been developed by the Department of Health.

Different countries have set different levels of RDAs, and have included slightly different ranges of nutrients. This means that the information given on nutritional labels of imported products may not conform to that on home produced foods. This should not be a cause of concern to the vast majority of people, for whom the RDAs are intended as broad guidelines.

In the United Kingdom RDAs have been established for vitamin A, vitamin B_1 (thiamin), vitamin B_2 (riboflavin), vitamin B_3 (niacin), vitamin C (ascorbic acid), vitamin D, calcium, iron and protein.

The RDAs are recommendations for healthy people only. Special nutrient needs for problems like premature birth, infections, chronic disease or the use of medication, stress, cigarette smoking, or some inherited metabolic disorders require special dietary attention. These conditions will not be covered by the RDAs. It is also very important to remember that each person's nutritional requirements will vary considerably with age, sex and level of mental and physical activity. In certain cases, for example where a nutrient is particularly important for pregnant or lactating women, a specific RDA has been established for the relevant group of individuals, but in other cases we must each make sure that we understand how all the various nutrients function so that we can take control of our own health.

Another limitation of the RDAs is how they are derived. Many of the recommendations are based on the amount required to reverse classical nutrient deficiency symptoms. For instance, the RDA for vitamin B_2 is based on the amount needed to correct a skin disorder that develops as a result of a deficiency of this vitamin. The vitamin's role in other disorders is often not considered because little information is available. When information is scarce recommendations are based on the quantities consumed by apparently healthy individuals.

Many experts now believe that the secrets of health are contained in the balanced diet. The foundation of this diet is the Four Food Groups. The vegetable-fruit group, the grain group, the milk group, and the meat-dried beans and peas group comprise this foundation. Although this diet implies solid nutrition, it often falls short of its mark. When poor choices are made or when the processing or preparation of these foods is

Table 2 Estimated Safe and Adequate Daily Dietery Intakes of Additional Nutrients

Age (years)	Vitamins			Trace elements							Electrolytes		
	Vitamin K (μg)	Biotin (μg)	Pantothenic acid (mg)	Copper (mg)	Manganese (mg)	Fluoride (mg)	Chromium (mg)	Selenium (mg)	Molybdenum (mg)		Sodium (mg)	Potassium (mg)	Chloride (mg)
0–0.5	12	35	2	0.5–0.7	0.5–0.7	0.1–0.5	0.01–0.04	0.01–0.04	0.03–0.06		115–350	350–925	275–700
0.5–1	10–20	50	3	0.7–1.0	0.7–1.0	0.2–1.0	0.02–0.06	0.02–0.06	0.04–0.08		250–750	425–1275	400–1200
1–3	15–30	65	3	1.0–1.5	1.0–1.5	0.5–1.5	0.02–0.08	0.02–0.08	0.05–0.1		325–975	550–1650	500–1500
4–6	20–40	85	3–4	1.5–2.0	1.5–2.0	1.0–2.5	0.03–0.12	0.03–0.12	0.06–0.15		450–1350	775–2325	700–2100
7–10	30–60	120	4–5	2.0–2.5	2.0–3.0	1.5–2.5	0.05–0.2	0.05–0.2	0.1 –0.3		600–1800	1000–3000	925–2775
11+	50–100	100–200	4–7	2.0–3.0	2.5–5.0	1.5–2.5	0.05–0.2	0.05–0.2	0.15–0.5		900–2700	1525–4575	1400–4200
Adults	70–140	100–200	4–7	2.0–3.0	2.5–5.0	1.5–4.0	0.05–0.2	0.05–0.5	0.15–0.5		1100–3300	1875–5625	1700–5100

*Because there is less information on which to base allowances, these figures are not given in the main table of the RDA and are provided here in the form of ranges of recommended intakes.

questionable, the nutrient content of the diet suffers.

Meeting nutrient needs through diet alone can be blocked by other lifestyle habits. People skip meals, snack, diet, and eat away from home. Taste and cost have always been significant factors in food choices and now convenience contributes to our eating habits. For those people who diet, have irregular eating habits skip meals, or choose poorly from food selections available, supplementation might be wise.

Marginal Deficiencies

Marginal deficiences are the middle ground between optimal nutritional status and the classical nutrient deficiency diseases. Scurvy or pellagra are actually the final stages of a nutrient deficiency and reflect months or years of poor dietary intake. Marginal deficiencies are difficult to detect since their symptoms are not specific. They often go undetected while their consequences undermine the quality of life.

Marginal deficiencies have been found in the elderly, pregnant women, and alcoholics. In one study, school children who consumed diets low in zinc were shorter in stature than children who consumed an adequate diet. Marginal deficiencies are found in a substantial number of hospitalised patients. Poor nutrition during illness can weaken the body's defence system, increase susceptibility to infection, and hamper the healing process. Vague discomfort and pain in the muscles, weakness, and ulcers in the elderly have been linked to marginal deficiencies of vitamin C. Increased susceptibility to colds and flu are more likely when people consume a diet that is marginally deficient in any one of a number of nutrients, including iron, zinc, vitamin A, vitamin B_{12}, vitamin B_6, and folic acid. When people consume a thiamin (vitaimin B_1) deficient diet, they report depression, anxiety, and nausea well before the appearance of signs of beriberi or tissue damage. Marginal deficiencies of vitamin C, thiamin, or riboflavin (vitamin B_2) can cause personality changes that include hypochondria, hysteria, and some emotional disorders.

Many degenerative diseases have been mistakenly thought to be the natural consequence of ageing. They are now suspected to be preventable through a lifetime of healthy habits.

Individuals At Risk Of Vitamin And Mineral Deficiencies

Several groups of people might benefit from vitamin-mineral supplements. These groups can be classified into three general categories:

- The first category is composed of people in specific groups, such as infants, adolescents, menstruating women, pregnant and breast-feeding women, the elderly, and people with chronic illness.
- People who negatively affect their nutritional well-being, such as alcoholics or cigarette smokers, people on long-term medications, and people under stress or with poor eating habits make up the second category.
- People who are on certain dietary programmes, such as the dieters, the strict vegetarians, and the food faddists compose the third category.

Supplements In Perspective

Nutrient-poor diets are common. Even when compared to the RDAs, a set of guidelines with limited usefulness when assessing individual dietary adequacy, many people's diets are lacking in several vitamins and minerals. Supplements cannot substitute for a nutritious and wholesome diet. Many substances in foods, other than vitamins and minerals, promote health and protect against disease. Compounds called "indoles" are found in some vegetables and appear to protect against certain forms of cancer. Some substances in garlic might lower blood cholesterol levels and prevent heart disease. These substances are not found in the supplements.

Supplements will not provide immunity from disease or prevent premature ageing in a body that is otherwise unhealthy, but they are an economical and practical means of ensuring adequate nutrition.

While supplements can have a useful place, it is also important to understand the nutritional value of all the foods we consume. In the case of many pre-packed foods this information is easily available on the label. Every individual should make a habit of reading labels, assessing their own personal nutritional status and supplementing accordingly. (*Figure 1, Page 16*).

Figure 1

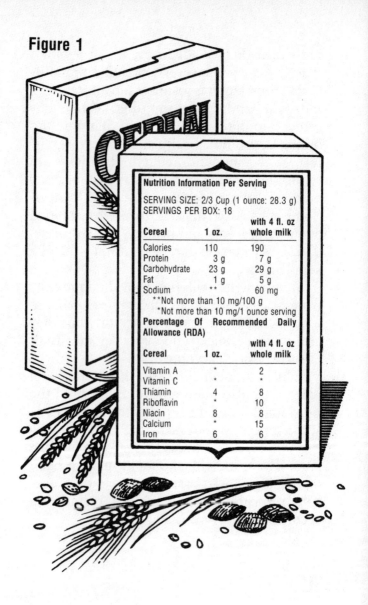

Nutrition Information Per Serving

SERVING SIZE: 2/3 Cup (1 ounce: 28.3 g)
SERVINGS PER BOX: 18

Cereal	1 oz.	with 4 fl. oz whole milk
Calories	110	190
Protein	3 g	7 g
Carbohydrate	23 g	29 g
Fat	1 g	5 g
Sodium	**	60 mg

**Not more than 10 mg/100 g
*Not more than 10 mg/1 ounce serving

Percentage Of Recommended Daily Allowance (RDA)

Cereal	1 oz.	with 4 fl. oz whole milk
Vitamin A	*	2
Vitamin C	*	*
Thiamin	4	8
Riboflavin	*	10
Niacin	8	8
Calcium	*	15
Iron	6	6

2

General Questions On Supplements

1. What Vitamin-Mineral Supplement Is The Best?

Vitamin and mineral needs vary widely from one individual to another. The following guidelines are designed to guarantee safety and economy when choosing an all-purpose vitamin-mineral supplement.

- Choose the multiple vitamin-mineral supplements, rather than an assortment of individual nutrients, unless they have been prescribed by a doctor. A multiple vitamin-mineral programme should include vitamins (the fat-soluble vitamins A, D, and E, and the water-soluble vitamins B_1, B_2, niacin, B_6, B_{12}, folacin, pantothenic acid, biotin, and vitamin C) and minerals (calcium, magnesium, iron, iodine, zinc, copper, manganese, chromium, selenium, and molybdenum).

- Choose preparations that provide approximately 100% of the RDAs for all the vitamins and minerals included in the formula.
- Avoid preparations that contain unrecognised or questionable nutrients, such as vitamin B_{15}, or nutrients in minute amounts. These inclusions do not increase the benefits of the preparation, but usually increase the cost.

2. Are High Doses Of Vitamins Or Minerals Harmful To My Health?

Some nutrients are toxic in high doses while others have a wide margin of safety. For example, the advised daily intake of vitamin B_6 is 2 mg. When the vitamin is taken in amounts between 500 mg and 2,000 mg nerve damage can result. Other B vitamins, such as niacin, pantothenic acid, and vitamin B_1, might be toxic in very large doses. Some other vitamins and minerals that can be toxic in very large doses are vitamin D, vitamin A, vitamin K, iron, copper, calcium, chromium, selenium, and zinc.

3. Are There Advantages To Taking Individual Vitamin Or Mineral Supplements Instead Of A Multiple?

Nutritional requirements vary widely from one individual to another. A complete multiple vitamin-mineral supplement provides most of the vitamins and minerals in a most convenient form; but individual supplements can be tailored to personal needs. For example, a pregnant woman might need extra iron and folic acid, someone on a diuretic medication for hypertension might need additional magnesium, or the female athlete might need extra vitamin B_2.

No single tablet or capsule provides all the nutrients in levels adequate to meet the RDA. The tablet would be the size of a golf ball. Either one or more nutrients is missing, or some nutrients are included in less than optimal amounts. If a single-dose multiple is used, you might want to supplement it with individual nutrients. Personalise the vitamin-mineral intake to meet your requirements as affected by medications, disease, stress, individual variation, or other factors.

4. Do I Need To Take A Supplement That Contains Both Vitamins And Minerals?

The body requires over 40 essential nutrients from the diet. All of these nutrients, both vitamins and minerals, are important in the healthy functioning of the body.

Besides their individual importance, the nutrients work as teams. Vitamin B_1 might have a specific role in the breakdown and release of energy from protein, carbohydrate, and fat, but it is useless without ample amounts of vitamin B_2, niacin, biotin, manganese, and several other nutrients. Bones require not only calcium for growth and maintenance but also vitamin D, magnesium, and phosphorus. If the preparation is labelled as a multiple vitamin, no minerals are present.

5. What Is The Difference Between Gm, Mg, And Mcg?

The gram (gm) is a metric unit of weight, equal to 1/28th of an ounce (28 grams = 1 ounce). A milligram (mg) is 1/1000th of a gram; a microgram (sometimes written μg) is 1/1000th of a milligram.

6. Which Vitamins Are Best, Synthetic Or Natural?

In most cases, there is little difference between synthetic and natural vitamins. Vitamins do not exist alone or apart from food unless they are synthesised in the laboratory or are extracted from food. In the latter case, they are exposed to chemical solvents during both their removal from the original food source and their concentration into tablets, capsules, or pills. What began as natural ends up as a highly refined and processed product. In many cases, the word "natural" is used on a vitamin or mineral supplement to indicate that the product is free from preservatives and additives.

Little scientific evidence exists to justify the use of natural over synthetic for most vitamins. Studies show the synthetic forms to be as effective as natural forms in the treatment and prevention of disease and the maintenance of health.

There are exceptions to this rule. Limited reseach does suggest that the natural form of vitamin E might have greater biological activity than the synthetic form of the vitamin. The natural yeast forms of selenium and chromium might have greater activity and safety than the inorganic forms.

7. What Is Chelation?

A chelated mineral is a mineral that is attached to another compound such as an amino acid. The term gluconate might appear after the name of the mineral to indicate that the mineral is chelated. For example, zinc gluconate is a chelated mineral. Chelation is the process of binding a mineral to another compound.

8. Are Chelated Minerals Better Than Regular Minerals?

The argument in favour of chelated minerals states that chelation improves the absorption and utilisation of the mineral. The attached amino acid carries the mineral across the intestinal lining into the blood system. Chelation, however, forms a weak bond that is easily broken in the acidic environment of the stomach. The benefits of chelation are more theory than fact. Chelated minerals, such as zinc gluconate, have one benefit; they are less irritating to the stomach and intestinal lining than mineral salts (e.g. zinc sulphate).

More important to its absorption than chelation is the circumstance under which a supplement is taken. Most vitamins and minerals are better absorbed if taken with a meal.

9. Should I Take Time-Released Vitamins?

The theory behind time-released vitamins makes sense. In reality they are probably no more effective than any other supplements.

The time-released supplements were designed to slow the release of vitamins in the intestine, increase the absorption, and reduce the dramatic fluctuations in blood levels. However, because vitamins are absorbed at specific places in the intestines, their release must be at the right moment or they will pass undigested in the stool. In a study, when time-released or regular niacin was given to patients with high blood cholesterol, the regular niacin supplement was more effective at lowering blood cholesterol and other fats than was the time-released tablet.

10. What Are Buffered Vitamins?

Some vitamins are acidic and might upset the body's acid/base balance when taken in large amounts. A buffer can be added to the supplement to counteract this acidity. "Ascorbate" is a form of buffered vitamin C.

11. Do Vitamins Or Minerals Lose Their Potency When Stored For Long Periods Of Time?

Vitamins can lose their potency over time or if not stored in a cool, dark area with the cap securely fastened. Most supplements include an expiry date on the label to protect against losses in vitamin potency. Minerals are the basic elements that comprise rocks. Even if the tablets disintegrate into a powder, their mineral content remains unchanged. If, however, minerals are combined with vitamins, the supplement must be treated as any vitamin supplement.

12. Do Supplements Increase Appetite?

Some people claim that supplements of the vitamin B complex increase appetite. Although this might be caused by a direct effect of the vitamins on the lining of the stomach, no scientific evidence exists to show that supplements increase appetite.

13. Are Chewable Vitamins Safe For Children?

Some brands of chewable vitamins contain sugars that might cause tooth decay. Sweetened vitamins can seem like sweets, which can result in excess consumption of some potentially toxic nutrients. Read the label and maintain intake at an appropriate dose.

3

Questions On Vitamins

14. What Is An Antioxidant?

Antioxidants are substances produced by the body or drawn from the diet that neutralise destructive compounds that might cause premature ageing, cancer, heart disease, and other degenerative diseases. Examples of dietary antioxidants are selenium, vitamin E, vitamin A, and vitamin C.

15. What Is A Free Radical?

Free radicals are highly reactive substances that result from cigarette smoke, air pollution, radiation, or incomplete breakdown of fats and protein in the body. Peroxides and superoxides formed from oxygen are also free radicals. A free radical can attack fats in the body, rupture cell membranes, and release harmful substances into the surrounding cells. Irreversible damage results and cell function is either altered or the cell dies. A strong antioxidant defence system might prevent damage from free radicals.

16. Is There A Difference Between Vitamin A From Fish Liver Oils, Retinoic Acid, And Beta-Carotene?

There are two basic categories of vitamin A: the preformed or active form called retinol or retinal, and the provitamin called the carotenoids, of which beta-carotene is the most common. The preformed vitamin A is found in fish liver oils and liver. The provitamin is found in plants and must be converted to the preformed vitamin once it enters the body. Despite differences in food sources and potencies, all forms of vitamin A are effective in the maintenance of healthy skin and eyes and might help prevent some types of cancer.

17. I Have Heard Vitamin A Can Be Toxic At High Levels. How Much Is Too Much?

The adult RDA for vitamin A is 750 μg, which is the amount of vitamin A in one small carrot or a serving of cooked broccoli. Retinol, the active form of the vitamin found in liver, fish liver oils, and in some supplements, in doses of as much as twenty times this amount can cause nausea, vomiting, joint and abdominal pain, bone abnormalities, hair loss, and liver damage. Children should not consume more than their RDA of retinol. The vitamin A in vegetables is called beta-carotene. No toxic symptoms, other than a yellowing of the skin, have been reported from this form of the vitamin.

18. Will The B Complex Give Me Energy?

No vitamin or mineral will provide energy directly. The energy in food is measured in "calories." The only substances in food that provide calories are protein, carbohydrates (sugar and starch), and fat. Vitamins and minerals do not contain calories or energy.

The B vitamins, as well as cobalt, copper, iron, magnesium, manganese, phosphorus, potassium, and zinc, are necessary for the extraction of energy. In this way, they are secondary providers of energy. However, consuming more B vitamins than the body needs will not give an added energy boost.

19. What Is Meant By The Term "Nutrient-Dense"?

Nutrient-dense foods are those foods that provide a high amount of one or more vitamins or minerals for a low amount of calories. Fresh vegetables, fruits, whole grain breads and cereals, nonfat dairy foods, dried beans and peas, and lean meats, chicken, and fish are considered nutrient-dense foods. If these foods are cooked in oil or butter, their nutrient density declines because of the increased calories supplied by the fat.

20. What Is The Difference Between Niacin And Niacinamide?

Niacin is a general term for two compounds: nicotinic acid and niacinamide (also called nicotinamide). Nicotinic acid in large doses might cause flushing of the skin; however, niacinamide does not cause flushing.

21. Why Do Supplements Not Provide More Folic Acid?

A deficiency of folic acid or of vitamin B_{12} causes similar symptoms, including anaemia, fatigue, and irritability. If a person is deficient in both vitamins and takes large doses of folic acid, the deficiency symptoms will subside and the underlying vitamin B_{12} deficiency will go undetected. Because prolonged deficiency of vitamin B_{12} can cause irreversible nerve damage, experts advise limiting supplemental folic acid to 400 mcg. (or μg) for adults and 800 mcg. for pregnant women.

22. What Is The Vitamin C Complex?

The term "vitamin C complex" is used by vitamin manufacturers to describe any supplement containing vitamin C (ascorbic acid), various other related compounds such as bioflavonoids, and rose hips. No standardisation exists for this term, so the type and amount of substances contained in a product will vary from one manufacturer to another.

23. What Are Bioflavonoids?

Though not a vitamin the bioflavonoids are a family of compounds that, in conjunction with vitamin C, might help strengthen capillary walls, reduce capillary breakage and leakage, and help prevent varicose veins and haemorrhoids. Evidence suggests that bioflavonoids also prevent bruising and damage to artery walls from free radical attack. No deficiency symptoms of bioflavonoids have been reported in humans or animals.

24. Will Vitamin C Prevent And Cure The Common Cold?

Vitamin C probably will not prevent the common cold, but it might minimise the symptoms associated with it. White blood cells, responsible for fighting infection, show increased activity when exposed to vitamin

C in the laboratory. This shows that a reduction in the severity of cold symptoms might be caused by vitamin C. Evidence does support this theory and shows that vitamin C, taken before or at the earliest signs of a cold, might reduce both the severity and duration of infection.

While moderate doses of vitamin C have been associated with increased resistance to colds and infections, in gram doses this water-soluble vitamin might inhibit the body's natural defence system and reduce its resistance to infections.

25. Can I Get Enough Vitamin D From The Sun?

Vitamin D is manufactured in the presence of sunlight by specialised cells in the skin. If a person is exposed to ample sunlight, this vitamin is not needed in the diet. The manufacture of vitamin D is restricted, however, by anything that limits the amount of sunlight reaching the skin.

26. What Foods Are High In Vitamin D?

The vitamin D content of egg yolks, butter, and liver varies and depends on the vitamin content of the foods the animals consumed. Vitamin D-fortified milk is the only reliable dietary source other than cod liver oil. Other milk products, such as yogurt and cheese, are not fortified and are not considered reliable sources of vitamin D.

Vitamin D is a fat-soluble vitamin and daily sources are not necessary since the vitamin is stored in the body. Large doses can be toxic and intake in adults should be restricted to the RDA of 2.5 μg unless otherwise directed by a physician. Children and infants are susceptible to toxic reactions and should not consume more than their RDA of 7.5 μg for vitamin D.

27. Why Do People Need Vitamin E?

Vitamin E is an antioxidant that protects fats in the body and the diet from destruction and rancidity. Free radicals taken into the body react with fats and this reaction causes cell damage. Vitamin E can deactivate these free radicals and stop the damage. Vitamin E protects against lung damage caused by air pollution, tissue damage from radiation exposure, tumour growth, the destruction of healthy tissue during chemotherapy, and the destruction of vitamin A.

Vitamin E also assists cells, especially those of the heart and muscles, in the absorption and use of oxygen; improves neurological and visual problems in older persons; protects red blood cells from premature destruction; and prevents some forms of anaemia. Vitamin E might be important in the treatment or prevention of cystic fibrosis, chronic liver disease, intermittent claudication, elevated blood cholesterol levels, oxygen deprivation in premature infants, muscular dystrophy, and sickle cell anaemia.

28. Since Vitamin E Is A Fat-Soluble Vitamin, Can Large Doses Be Toxic?

Studies in animals show that a large intake of vitamin E might impair the absorption of vitamins A and K. Toxic symptoms seen in animals include retarded growth, anaemia, poor blood clotting, and slowed bone formation. No toxic symptoms have been reported in humans.

29. What Is The Difference Between D-alpha Tocopherol And Mixed Tocopherols?

Vitamin E is a family of vitamins called the tocopherols, of which d-alpha-tocopherol is the most biologically active form. The other naturally occurring tocopherols include beta-, gamma-, and delta-tocopherols. The synthetic forms of vitamin E, like dl-alpha tocopherol, are attempts to duplicate the natural forms of the vitamin. A preparation that contains mixed tocopherols includes all of the natural forms of vitamin E and more closely resembles the vitamin E found in foods. An excellent source of mixed tocopherols is wheat germ oil.

30. If My Diet Is High In Vegetable Oils, Do I Need More Vitamin E?

Vitamin E protects unsaturated fats from destruction and rancidity. Vegetable fats are primarily unsaturated and as their intake increases the requirement for vitamin E increases. To reduce the risk of developing some types of cancer, the consumption of fats including polyunsaturated fats, should be kept to a minimum.

31. Does Processing Of Foods Affect Their Vitamin E Content?

Substantial loss of vitamin E occurs during the processing and bleaching of oils, flours, and other vegetable foods. These foods increase the daily requirement but supply little vitamin E. Cold pressed vegetable oils and the oils found naturally in nuts, seeds, and other foods contain ample amounts of vitamin E.

32. Does Vitamin E Improve Fertility?

In the 1920's, studies showed that vitamin E prevented infertility and degeneration of the sex organs in rats. Animal research has continued to show an association between a vitamin E deficiency and sexual dysfunction. No association has been found between human reproduction or sexual performance and vitamin E.

4

Questions On Minerals

33. Who Needs Calcium Supplements?

Although everyone requires calcium, the devastating effects of a deficiency are most pronounced in women. One out of four women develops osteoporosis and many painful bone fractures each year are attributed to osteoporosis. Characterised by a progressive shortening of stature and curvature of the spine, lower back pain, and increased risk of broken or cracked bones, osteoporosis often can be prevented or the process slowed if a person consumes adequate calcium and maintains a regular exercise programme. Low calcium intake is also linked to deterioration of bone that supports the teeth, and high blood pressure in both men and women.

34. When Should I Start Taking Calcium Supplements?

Adequate calcium intake is important throughout life. Bone growth is rapid through childhood and the teen years. The teen years through to the twenties are a time for continued calcium deposition that increases bone density. Calcium intake during these two periods is most critical for optimal bone growth and maturation. Bone growth reaches a peak when a person is about 30 years old to 35 years old. After this peak, bone density begins to decline and unless calcium intake equals or exceeds calcium losses, the bones begin to dissolve.

35. How Much Calcium Should I Take?

Evidence shows that a calcium intake that meets the RDA (500 mg) may not be sufficient to halt the progress of osteoporosis and that intakes of 1,000 mg or more are necessary.

Calcium intake becomes even more vital for women after menopause when bone degeneration increases as oestrogen levels decline. A daily intake of 1,000 mg to 1,500 mg, either from dietary sources or supplements, should reduce bone loss in women not on oestrogen therapy. To ensure calcium absorption and use, adequate vitamin D is necessary from exposure to sunlight or ingestion of foods rich in vitamin D.

36. How Can I Tell If My Diet Is Low In Calcium?

Large scale surveys show that many people, especially adults, are not consuming their recommended amounts of calcium. If a person does not consume a minimum of three servings of milk, yogurt, dark green leafy vegetables, or other foods high in calcium each day, the diet might not be adequate in this mineral.

37. What Is The Best Calcium Supplement?

The best supplemental sources of calcium are calcium lactate, calcium carbonate, and calcium gluconate. The absorption of calcium lactate is slightly better than the other supplements. The amount of calcium in each tablet of calcium gluconate or lactate, however, is small and as many as 6 tablets must be taken to meet the RDA of 500 mg calcium. In contrast, calcium carbonate is well absorbed, is a concentrated source of the mineral, and fewer tablets are needed to meet the RDA.

38. Can A Person Consume Too Much Calcium?

Information on the effects of a calcium overdose in humans is scarce. A daily intake of from 1,000 mg to 1,500 mg has been recommended for adults and for post-menopausal women.

39. Are Dolomite And Bone Meal Good Sources Of Calcium?

Samples of both dolomite and bone meal have been found to contain trace amounts of toxic metals, such as lead.

40. Will Calcium Supplements Increase My Chances Of Developing Kidney Stones?

Calcium from the diet or supplements is a safe and essential nutrient unless individuals have a metabolic disorder that places them at risk of kidney stones.

41. Should I Take Magnesium With My Calcium Supplement?

Calcium and magnesium are both essential minerals in bone formation and maintenance and in proper functioning of blood vessels and of nerves. Diets without many whole-grain cereals or green vegetables are often low in these two minerals and a deficiency of both is associated with high blood pressure, atherosclerosis, or heart disease. When the calcium intake is adequate but the intake of magnesium is low, blood calcium levels will drop and remain low until magnesium intake is increased.

42. Do I Need Extra Calcium If I Am On A High Protein Diet Or Use Protein Powders?

Calcium requirements increase with a high protein intake. A reduction of protein, rather than additional supplements of calcium, is suggested.

Many of us regularly consume two to three times more protein than the body needs. A high protein diet increases the loss of calcium in the urine. This elevates the daily calcium requirement to replace these losses. The extra protein is wasted, places a stress on both the liver and kidneys, and contributes to a calcium deficiency.

43. Why Do I Need Chromium?

Chromium is a trace mineral essential for the maintenance of normal blood sugar and heart and blood vessel function. A chromium deficiency resembles the symptoms of diabetes and these symptoms sometimes disappear with chromium supplementation. Chromium is linked to heart disease from evidence that a chromium deficiency raises blood levels of cholesterol. When chromium is added to the diet, levels of cholesterol decline.

44. How Much Chromium Is Enough?

The American diet contains only 25 mcg/ 1000 calories. Since it is advised by some experts that chromium consumption should be between 50 mcg and 200 mcg per day, a person would have to eat 8,000 calories to obtain the upper recommended limit. A person who consumes less than 2,000 calories or consumes a diet high in refined and processed foods would not meet even the lower end of the scale for chromium. Chromium deficiency does occur and marginal chromium intake is common in the United States. This might contribute to the high incidence of diabetes and heart disease in that country. To avoid any unnecessary risk, particularly if you tend to eat more processed and refined foods, the diet should contain the daily recommendations for chromium. There is no evidence that a greater intake is necessary for optimal health and an excess can be toxic.

45. What Is GTF?

Chromium functions in our blood sugar regulation as a part of a biologically active compound called Glucose Tolerance Factor (GTF). GTF is manufactured in the body from niacin, a few amino acids, and three atoms of chromium or it can be obtained from the diet. It is the best absorbed and utilised form of the chromium. If brewer's yeast is grown on chromium-rich soil, it is an excellent source of GTF chromium.

46. Can A Copper Deficiency Cause Heart Disease?

A copper deficiency has been linked to both heart disease and abnormal glucose tolerance, which is a warning sign of diabetes. Copper is involved in the manufacture of cholesterol in the liver, but how a copper deficiency affects this process is poorly understood. Copper deficiency damages the artery walls, which are then more prone to breaking. This would explain the increased death rate from cardiac rupture observed in animals with copper deficiency.

47. What Are Good Dietary Sources Of Copper?

Good dietary sources of copper include liver, kidneys, shellfish, nuts, whole grain breads and cereals, raisins, cocoa, dried beans and peas, and the dark green leafy vegetables.

48. What Are The Signs Of Iron Deficiency?

Iron is part of haemoglobin, a protein molecule in red blood cells that binds to oxygen and carries it to all the cells in the body. When the diet is low in iron, the body cannot produce haemoglobin and the body's cells are deprived of oxygen. The condition is called anaemia and its symptoms are irritability, fatigue, poor concentration, thinning of the fingernails, increased colds and infections, a decline in work performance, and being out of breath after climbing stairs or a brief walk.

49. Who Is At Risk Of Iron Deficiency?

Iron deficiency is a very common nutritional deficiency and its prevalence might range up to 50% in some segments of the population. It affects primarily women, pregnant women, infants, children, teenagers, athletes, the elderly, low-income groups, and minorities. The average diet provides about 6 mg of iron/1,000 calories. An average calorie intake of 1,400 to 1,600 will thus not even meet the RDA for men, let alone for women. Many experts agree that a typical modern Western diet cannot meet the daily iron requirements of at least 10 mg.

50. What Is The Best Iron Supplement?

Iron is found in two forms, ferric and ferrous. The ferrous form is better absorbed than the ferric form. Ferrous sulphate can be irritating to the stomach and intestines and can cause nausea, heartburn, and either diarrhoea or constipation in some people. These side effects can be minimised by increasing the dose gradually over several

days. Ferrous fumarate, succinate, and gluconate are absorbed well and are good
sources of iron.

51. What Foods Or Supplements Interfere With Iron Absorption?

Several foods, medications, and supplements impair iron absorption. These
include the tannin in tea and coffee, eggs,
antacids, the antibiotic tetracycline, phosphorus and phosphate additives, some preservatives, phytates in unleavened whole
grain breads, oxalates in spinach and chard,
and soy products. The effect of these factors
on iron absorption varies. For instance,
orange juice increases the absorption of iron
from eggs and whole grain breads, but the
poor absorption of iron from bread is further
reduced if it is eaten with an egg and no
juice.

52. How Can I Improve Iron Intake?

General guidelines for increasing iron
absorption are to consume a vitamin C-rich

food with iron, include a small quantity of meat, fish, or chicken with generous servings of vegetables and grains in a meal, and avoid drinking either tea or coffee with meals. Additionally, increase consumption of iron-rich foods and take a daily supplement of iron if recommended by a doctor.

53. I Read That Foods Cooked In An Iron Pan Are A Good Source Of Iron. Is This True?

Iron pots improve the iron content of most foods. The iron leaches from the pot into the food during the cooking. The longer the food is in contact with the pot, and the more acid that is in the food (e.g. tomato sauce) the greater the iron content of the final product. Seasoning cast iron pots (sealing off the pores of a pot with oil) will reduce the amount of iron that leaches into the food.

54. How Would I Know If I Were Deficient In Magnesium?

The signs of magnesium deficiency are subtle and a marginal deficiency can go undetected indefinitely. Weakness, mental confusion, personality changes, muscle cramps, loss of appetite, nausea, tooth decay, lack of coordination, stomach problems, loss of hair, swollen gums, skin sores, and heart disease can be symptoms of mild to severe magnesium deficiency. Diuretic medications used in the treatment of hypertension can precipitate a magnesium deficiency, as can alcohol, tetracycline, and some other medications.

55. Why Do I Need Manganese? How Can I Tell If My Diet Is Adequate In This Mineral?

Manganese is important in the breakdown of protein, fats, and carbohydrates for energy. It is also needed for normal digestion and the production of protein in the body. The blood will not clot after an injury, bones do not develop correctly, and the immune system fails to function at optimum levels without an adequate supply of manganese. Dietary sources of manganese include liver, kidney, lettuce, spinach, meat, whole grain breads and cereals, dried beans and peas, and nuts. Large amounts of manganese might reduce iron absorption and impair red blood cell formation.

56. Why Do I Need Molybdenum? What Are Good Dietary Sources Of This Mineral?

Molybdenum is an important component of iron metabolism and red blood cell formation. Good dietary sources include whole grain breads and cereals, meat, dried beans and peas, and offal meats.

57. I Work In A Hot Environment And Am Concerned That I Might Be Losing Excess Potassium When I Perspire. Should I Take Salt Or Potassium Tablets?

The body is very efficient at conserving minerals and little potassium or sodium is lost through the skin. Instead, these minerals become more concentrated in the body as more and more water is lost as perspiration. To replace potassium or sodium prior to replacing water losses could result in over-concentration of these minerals in the body, heart arrhythmias, and organ damage. The potassium lost by perspiring can be replaced easily by the inclusion of vegetables and fruits in the daily diet. There is no need to replace sodium losses since the average modern diet is already high in sodium (salt) and excessive consumption of this mineral is linked to hypertension.

58. Why Did My Doctor Recommend I Take Potassium Tablets Along With My Blood Pressure Medication?

Some diuretic medications increase the excretion of potassium, and a deficiency can result unless a potassium supplement is taken. It is important to consult a doctor regarding prescription-strength potassium supplementation since not all diuretics deplete potassium and extra potassium when it is not needed might cause heart arrhythmias, kidney damage, and other adverse side effects.

59. I Thought Selenium Was A Toxic Mineral And Now I Hear It Is Essential To Health. Which Is True?

Selenium is both toxic and essential to health. In doses of several times the level considered safe and adequate, selenium can cause retarded growth, damage to eyes, hair loss, impaired bone formation, tooth decay, and increased risk of liver and heart disease.

Selenium is needed in small amounts as a component of an enzyme that protects the body from damage caused by oxygen, peroxides, and other free radicals. (Question 15) As an antioxidant, selenium protects the body against cell damage, some forms of cancer, and heart disease. The safe and adequate range for selenium is 50 mcg to 200 mcg. The suggested upper limit for selenium is 500 mcg/day.

60. Why Do I Need Zinc?

Zinc helps strengthen the body's defence against infection, colds, and possibly cancer. People with a reduced resistance to infection often have low levels of zinc in their blood.

When zinc is added to the diet, resistance to disease improves. Inadequate zinc intake also can reduce the taste sensation, retard growth, and cause hair loss. Large doses of zinc (above 100 mg) might inhibit the immune system, elevate blood levels of cholesterol, and increase risks of infection and disease.

61. What Is The Difference Between Zinc Gluconate And Zinc Sulphate?

Both of these forms of zinc are equally well absorbed and used by the body. However, sulphate is more acidic and can be irritating to the stomach and the intestinal lining. If you experience nausea, diarrhoea, constipation, heartburn, or distension switch to zinc gluconate or take zinc sulphate with meals.

62. Why Is Zinc Added To Some Calcium Supplements?

Most of the factors that cause increased excretion of calcium, such as a high fibre diet, also increase zinc losses and it is thus possible that a diet low in one would be low in the other.

Limited evidence shows that zinc might be involved in the transportation of calcium across the intestinal lining and might be necessary for optimal absorption of calcium.

63. Can Zinc Supplements Cause A Copper Deficiency?

The balance is very important when it comes to trace mineral absorption and metabolism. Zinc and copper provide an example of two minerals that are delicately balanced. When the ratio of zinc to copper is offset by the consumption of too much zinc, copper excretion increases, copper retention declines, and a copper deficiency can result.

5

Questions On Vitamins/Minerals And Specific Health Issues

64. Do I Need To Take A Vitamin B$_{12}$ Supplement If I Am A Vegetarian?

Vitamin B$_{12}$ is only found in foods from animal sources. If a plant food contains this vitamin it is from bacterial fermentation or contamination, as with some fermented soy products such as miso. If the diet does not contain eggs, dairy foods, or foods from animal sources then it will be low in vitamin B$_{12}$. Body stores can last from a few months to several years, but eventually symptoms of vitamin B$_{12}$ deficiency will develop. Anaemia, fatigue, poor concentration, irritability, headaches, or depression are the initial signs. If the deficiency is not treated, then irreversible nerve damage can result.

65. As A Vegetarian, Do I Need To Take A Zinc Supplement?

The high fibre diet, which interferes with the absorption of zinc, combined with a lack of zinc-rich meat in the diet might place a vegetarian at risk of zinc deficiency. If a person watches his or her calorie intake and consumes mostly fruits and vegetables rather than good dietary sources of zinc such as nuts, seeds, dried beans and peas, and whole grain breads and cereals, the likelihood of a low zinc intake in the vegetarian diet is increased. A daily intake of at least 10 mg is advised.

66. Can Rheumatoid Arthritis Be Treated With Diet?

The causes of rheumatoid arthritis are not well understood, but it is known that a well-nourished body is better equipped to combat infection and disease than a malnourished body. Deficiencies of folic acid, vitamin D, vitamin B_6, and iron have been found in patients with arthritis. Pain and stiffness are often improved when patients take a zinc supplement. The inflammation associated with rheumatoid arthritis might be caused, in part, by peroxides and other free radicals. The antioxidants, vitamin E and selenium, show promise in relieving the symptoms associated with inflammation. Calcium also might help to diminish symptoms.

67. I Am On A Low Sodium Diet. Should I Avoid Vitamins/ Minerals That Contain Sodium, Such As Sodium Ascorbate?

The sodium from sodium ascorbate is quite like any other source of dietary sodium and will contribute to the total day's intake. Approximately one-tenth of the tablet is sodium. This can total a substantial amount (1 gram) of sodium if a person takes a ten-gram dose. If sodium ascorbate is taken because it does not upset the stomach, try calcium ascorbate or the ascorbate with magnesium or potassium as a low-sodium alternative.

68. I Am A Senior Citizen. Should I Take Supplements?

The elderly are one of the most nutritionally vulnerable groups. Nutritional deficiencies might be more common than was originally thought since the ageing process can mask or overlap the recognised signs or symptoms of nutritional deficiencies.

Elderly people who do not take supplements can be low in vitamins A, E, C, B_1, B_2, B_{12}, folic acid, selenium, and chromium. These deficiencies are not as common when supplements are a part of the diet. For some nutrients such as vitamin C, the RDA might not be adequate to maintain optimal nutritional status in healthy older people and as much as twice the RDA or even more might be required for satisfactory intake. If a person is taking medication, is ill, or is under some stress a greater intake might be necessary.

69. I Drink Several Soft Drinks Each Day. Will This Affect My Health?

Soft drinks can contain as much as 150 calories per serving. If several servings are consumed each day, this can amount to a substantial proportion of the day's allotment of calories. If sugary foods comprise more than 10% of the diet, malnutrition becomes possible.

Both diet and regular soft drinks contain phosphates. A high phosphate intake can reduce calcium absorption, increase urinary excretion of calcium, and remove calcium from the bones. Over the years, this can contribute to osteoporosis and other degenerative bone diseases.

70. What Nutrients Might Be Lacking In A Fast Food Diet?

Fast foods, such as hamburgers, hot dogs, fried chicken, french fries, and soft drinks, are high in calories, fat (especially saturated fat), sodium, and sugar. Vitamins, minerals, and other nutrients that are low in these foods include fibre, vitamin A, vitamin C, folacin, biotin, pantothenic acid, copper, vitamin E, vitamin B_6, calcium, and magnesium. Other nutrient deficiencies associated with a high fat, low fibre diet include chromium, selenium, manganese, and molybdenum.

71. I Am A Cigarette Smoker. Do I Need To Take Vitamins?

Smoking is the number one risk factor for lung cancer. The vitamins and minerals that might protect against the development and growth of lung cancer are selenium, vitamin E, vitamin A and beta-carotene, and vitamin C. An adequate intake of vitamin A or carotene reduces the cancer risk even in people who smoke or chew tobacco. Smokers are two to three times more likely to show signs of vitamin C deficiency than non-smokers and a normal dietary intake might not be adequate to maintain the body stores of this vitamin in this population.

72. I Have A Drinking Problem. Am I At Risk Of Vitamin Or Mineral Deficiencies?

Excessive consumption of alcohol is a cause of many vitamin and mineral deficiencies. The poor eating habits that often accompany alcohol abuse is one reason for malnutrition. Even in the presence of adequate nutrient intake, excessive alcohol consumption might aggravate alcohol-induced tissue damage such as cirrhosis of the liver and reduced resistance to infection. Nutrient deficiencies associated with alcohol abuse include folic acid, vitamin B_1, vitamin A, vitamin B_2, niacin, vitamin C, vitamin B_6, vitamin B_{12}, magnesium, selenium, and zinc.

73. What Vitamins Or Minerals Do I Need If I Am Under Stress?

Nutrition and stress are closely related. While stressful times might deplete certain vitamins and minerals from the body, poor nutrition can reduce a person's ability to cope effectively with stress. Some nutrients, such as vitamin C, zinc, vitamin B_6, and vitamin A, are important in the maintenance of a healthy immune system, the body's defence against disease. Since stress affects the immune system, a person might need more of these nutrients. The body's stores of magnesium, the B vitamins, chromium, and vitamin C also tend to be low during times of stress.

74. Are There Vitamins Or Minerals I Should Take When Dieting?

If food intake is restricted to less than 2,000 calories, then it is advisable to take a daily multiple vitamin-mineral preparation.

75. Are There Vitamins Or Minerals That Protect Against Colds And Flu?

Nutrients that strengthen the immune system might help to protect against colds and disease. Vitamins and minerals that are associated with a healthy immune system include vitamin A and beta-carotene, vitamin B_1, vitamin B_2, niacin, vitamin B_6, biotin, folacin, pantothenic acid, vitamin C, vitamin D, vitamin E, iron, selenium, and zinc.

76. Will A High Fibre Diet Affect The Absorption Of Minerals?

Fibre in the diet is an aid in the prevention of heart disease, cancer, and diabetes. More than about 60 grams of fibre a day, however, can reduce the absorption of iron, zinc, calcium, magnesium, and phosphorus. If the daily diet contains several servings of whole grain breads and cereals, fresh fruits and vegetables, and legumes, there in no reason to consume added fibre from bran or other high fibre products.

77. Is It True That Zinc And Vitamin A Will Speed Wound Healing?

Zinc and vitamin A have been used effectively in wound healing and in the treatment of other skin lesions.

78. Are There Any Vitamins Or Minerals That Can Help In The Treatment of Acne?

Zinc and vitamin A have been used with some success in the treatment of acne and psoriasis. Acne is a complex disorder that requires the supervision of a doctor.

79. Is Premenstrual Syndrome (PMS) Caused By A Vitamin Or Mineral Deficiency?

Certain vitamins and minerals might reduce some of the symptoms of PMS. Vitamin B_6 might lessen the severity of headaches, water retention, bloating, depression, and also irritability associated with PMS. Vitamin E, vitamin A, magnesium, and zinc also may reduce symptoms of breast tenderness, acne, dizziness, or cravings for sweets.

80. Are There Any Vitamins Or Minerals That Help Treat Heart Disease Or Elevated Blood Cholesterol?

The B vitamins are important in the production and use of fats in the body. Some B vitamins, such as niacin, lower blood cholesterol levels. A vitamin B_6 deficiency can damage the artery wall and increase the risk of heart disease. Vitamin C plays a role in cholesterol synthesis and use, the maintenance of the artery lining, and, in some cases, reduces total cholesterol and increases HDL-cholesterol. Vitamins A and E also might protect the artery walls from damage and alter blood chemistry to discourage atherosclerosis. In contrast, vitamin D in large doses might encourage either the deposition of calcium into the arteries or platelet clumping. Either action would promote the development of atherosclerosis.

Adequate intake of minerals, including magnesium, chromium, zinc, copper, calcium, iodine, and iron are important in reducing both blood cholesterol and the risk of heart disease.

81. Are There Any Vitamins Or Minerals That Help Prevent Cancer?

Too much fat and too little fibre are the primary factors in the link between diet and cancer. Several vitamins and minerals also might play a role in cancer prevention. Adequate intakes of vitamin C, vitamin A, beta-carotene, vitamin E, zinc, and selenium are likely to reduce a person's risk of several types of cancer.

82. Are There Any Vitamins Or Minerals That Help Prevent Or Treat Diabetes?

Chromium might be of benefit in the treatment and prevention of diabetes. Chromium deficiency resembles glucose intolerance and, in some cases, the addition of chromium to the diet helps normalise blood sugar in hyperglycaemics and diabetics. Chromium supplementation also might help normalise blood sugar in people with hypoglycaemia. Diabetics often have problems with immune function, wound healing, and circulation in the extremities. Vitamin C might assist in the treatment of these conditions, especially since diabetics and people with elevated blood sugar are prone to marginal deficiencies of this vitamin.

83. Are There Any Minerals That Help Prevent Or Treat Hypertension (High Blood Pressure)?

Calcium supplementation lowers blood pressure in some hypertensives. A low intake of potassium in relationship to sodium is linked with elevated blood pressure. Potassium supplements are not recommended unless prescribed by a doctor, but the consumption of foods high in potassium and low in salt would result in a high ratio of potassium to sodium and might help reduce blood pressure.

The ratio of copper to zinc also might play a role in blood pressure regulation. When dietary intake of copper is high and zinc intake is low, blood pressure is more likely to be elevated.

Besides vitamins and minerals, a low-fat, high-fibre vegetarian diet also aids in the prevention and treatment of hypertension.

84. Are There Any Vitamins Or Minerals That Treat Or Prevent Hearing Problems?

A deficiency of vitamin D is found in some people with hearing impairment. Vitamin D might improve hearing by its effect on the bony tissues of the ear such as the cochlea. (*Figure 2*, *Page 69*) Whether supplementation with the vitamin would be of benefit in cases of deafness or hearing loss has not been well researched. When some people with hearing loss increase their intake of iodine, hearing improves. In both cases, supplementation would only benefit those who were already deficient in the nutrient.

Iodine and vitamin D can be toxic when taken in large amounts and intake greater than the RDA should be supervised by a doctor.

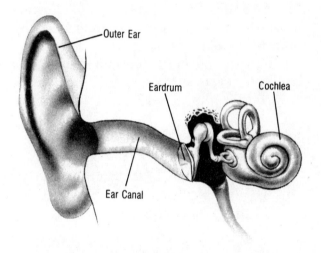

Figure 2.

Vitamin D might improve hearing by strengthening the inner bones of the ear, including the cochlea

85. Is There A Supplement I Can Take To Improve My Eyesight?

A vitamin B_2 deficiency can cause changes in the eye that can affect eyesight. One of the first symptoms of a vitamin A deficiency is difficulty in driving at night or seeing in dim light. If the vitamin A deficiency is not corrected, the disorder worsens and the eye becomes dry and distorted with further impairment in vision. Vitamin E also improves some visual defects. Chromium might play a role in the prevention of myopia and other eye disorders.

86. Are There Vitamins Or Minerals That Protect The Lungs From Damage Caused By Air Pollution Or Second Hand Cigarette Smoke?

Vitamin A (or beta-carotene) and vitamin E help protect lung tissue from damage caused by ozone in the air and irritants in smoke. Ozone might deplete the lung tissue of anti-oxidants and reduce the tissue's ability to defend itself against further damage. Other antioxidants such as selenium also might

provide protection against some environ-
mental pollutants.

87. Are There Any Vitamins Or Minerals That Will Help Me Lose Weight?

A diet that includes a wide range of nutrient-
dense foods and restricts the calorie intake,
combined with a regular exercise programme, is the only proven effective and
safe way to lose and maintain weight loss.

88. Which Nutrients, If Any, Prevent Premature Ageing?

Deficiencies of several vitamins and minerals are associated with premature ageing.
These include vitamin B_6, copper, folic acid,
vitamin B_{12}, vitamin E, and vitamin D. If
heart disease, osteoporosis, cancer, or
arthritis are classified as symptoms of
premature ageing this list of nutrients would
lengthen.

89. I Am Tired Much Of The Time. Could This Be A Vitamin Deficiency?

Tiredness or lethargy are both common symptoms of almost all nutrient deficiencies. Tiredness also can be a symptom of other lifestyle problems, and if it persists a doctor should be consulted regarding not only the possible nutrient deficiencies but also other underlying emotional or physical disorders.

90. What Vitamins Or Minerals Are Beneficial For Hair?

A diet that contains adequate amounts of all vitamins and minerals is essential for healthy hair. Without ample amounts of these nutrients, in particular, vitamin C, vitamin A, pantothenic acid, zinc, and copper, hair can become thin, dry, brittle, or lifeless.

91. What Vitamins Or Minerals Are Beneficial For Nails?

Nails become brittle, develop ridges, and crack easily when a person has an iron deficiency. A long-term deficiency results in spoon-shaped nails. Without an adequate intake of vitamin B_{12}, folic acid, copper, vitamin C, vitamin B_6, and other nutrients the oxygen-carrying capacity of the blood is reduced and nails are more likely to grow slowly, split, peel, or break.

92. What Vitamins Or Minerals Are Beneficial For Skin?

Poor dietary intake of one or more of the following will affect the softness, tone, colour, moisture, or strength of the skin: vitamin A, vitamin B_2, vitamin B_6, vitamin B_{12}, vitamin C, vitamin D, vitamin E, vitamin K, folic acid, pantothenic acid, niacin, biotin, iron, and zinc.

Questions On Miscellaneous Food Supplements

93. Will Choline Or Lecithin Improve Memory?

Some studies suggest supplementary choline might be effective in improving memory loss associated with ageing. Other studies show no improvement. Lecithin raises blood choline levels to a greater degree and for a longer duration than choline and is considered a type of "time-released" choline. However, increased blood levels of choline do not necessarily mean that memory and brain functioning will improve. Choline or lecithin taken in large amounts can cause acute gastrointestinal problems, depression, sweating, salivation, and loss of appetite.

94. Should I Take EPA To Prevent Heart Disease?

EPA (also called eicosapentaenoic acid or omega–3 fatty acid) is a type of fat found in fatty, cold-water fish such as mackerel and salmon. EPA lowers blood cholesterol and triglycerides, increases HDL-cholesterol, and reduces the risk of heart disease. Inclusion of fish in the diet will increase the intake of EPA or the fat can be taken in supplemental form.

95. I've Heard Garlic Will Prevent Heart Disease. Is This True?

Nothing will guarantee immunity from heart disease, but garlic might improve the odds. Garlic dissolves blood clots, inhibits clot formation, and lowers blood triglyceride and cholesterol levels. These are only a few of the beneficial effects of garlic in prevention and treatment of atherosclerosis and heart disease.

96. Will Phenylalanine Help Me Lose Weight?

Phenylalanine is an amino acid that has gained notoriety as a weight loss aid. Phenylalanine does stimulate the release of a hormone-like substance that plays a role in appetite regulation, but there is no evidence that phenylalanine affects long-term weight loss.

97. Does Acidophilus Protect Against Cancer?

People who consume yogurt that contains the bacteria called Lactobacillus acidophilus (L acidophilus) also tend to have a reduced incidence of colon cancer. Not all factory made yogurts contain L acidophilus. Many contain some other bacterias that are not as effective in lowering the risk for cancer. L acidophilus tablets are also a source of the bacteria. If supplements are used, moderation is suggested.

98. Is Lysine An Effective Treatment For Herpes?

Some studies show that lysine reduces the frequency and severity of herpes eruptions. The effectiveness of this amino acid in the treatment of herpes might depend on the maintenance of optimal blood levels of lysine. This requires a daily intake of as much as 1 gram or more of supplemental lysine to prevent recurrence. In large doses, lysine might interfere with the absorption of other amino acids.

99. Can Tryptophan Improve Sleep?

The amino acid tryptophan is the building block for a chemical called serotonin that regulates sleep and mood in the brain. Tryptophan, taken with a high-carbohydrate, low-protein snack, can improve the length and quality of sleep for some people. The amino acid also has proved beneficial for chronic insomniacs. The effect of long-term use of tryptophan has not been studied.

100. Where Can I Find Advice On Nutrition For My Personal Circumstances?

If you have any particular worries it is always best to consult your doctor. There are further books in this series giving more detailed advice on nutrition for children, the elderly, women, those suffering from stress, those wanting to lose weight and those concerned about their teeth, hair, nails, skin and bones.

Your Personalised Supplement Plan: A Worksheet

Read through the guidelines for choosing a vitamin-mineral supplement listed on pages 17–20. After identifying additional nutrients that might be useful or necessary for your specific concerns, use the worksheet below to tailor a supplement plan that is balanced, complete, and optimal for you.

Nutrient	Amount (mcg., mg., IU)	Nutrient	Amount (mcg., mg., IU)
Vitamin A or beta-carotene	_____	Pantothenic Acid	_____
Vitamin E	_____	Biotin	_____
Vitamin D	_____	Vitamin C	_____
Vitamin B_1 (thiamin)	_____	Calcium	_____
Vitamin B_2 (riboflavin)	_____	Chromium	_____
Niacin	_____	Iron	_____
Vitamin B_6	_____	Magnesium	_____
Vitamin B_{12}	_____	Selenium	_____
Folic Acid	_____	Zinc	_____

Glossary

Amino Acid: A building block of protein; over 20 amino acids are used by the body to form proteins in hair, skin, blood, and other tissues.

Anaemia: A reduction in the number, size, or colour of red blood cells; results in reduced oxygen-carrying capacity of the blood.

Antioxidant: A compound that protects other compounds or tissues from oxygen by reacting with oxygen.

Atherosclerosis: An accumulation of fat in the artery walls. The arteries become roughened and narrowed and blood flow is restricted. It is the underlying cause of heart attacks and strokes.

Beriberi: A disease caused by a deficiency

of thiamin and characterised by nerve disorders, weakness, mental disturbances, dermatitis, and heart failure.

Calorie: A measurement of heat. In nutrition, calorie refers to the quantity of energy contained in foods.

Carbohydrate: The starches and sugars in the diet.

Carotene: The form of vitamin A found in plants.

Chelate: To combine a metal with another compound.

Chemotherapy: The treatment of a disorder with medication.

Cholesterol: A fat-like substance found in animal fats and produced by the body.

Dermatitis: Inflammation of the skin that can be seen as a rash, sores, discolouration, eruptions, or ulcers.

Diabetes: A disorder in which the body's ability to use sugar is impaired because of inadequate production or utilisation of the hormone insulin.

Diuretic: A substance that increases the flow of urine.

Enzyme: A protein produced by the body that initiates and accelerates chemical reactions.

Free Radical: A highly reactive compound derived from air pollution, radiation, cigarette smoke, or the incomplete breakdown of proteins and fats; reacts with fats in cell membranes and changes their shape or function.

Glucose Tolerance Factor: A chromium-containing compound that enhances the function of insulin and helps regulate the glucose metabolism.

Haematocrit: The volume percent of red blood cells in whole blood.

Haemoglobin: The oxygen-carrying protein in red blood cells.

Haemorrhoids: Enlarged veins (varicose

veins) in the lower portion of the colon and surrounding the area of the anus.

Herpes: A skin disorder caused by a virus and characterised by pain and blisters.

Hormone: A chemical substance produced by a group of cells or an organ, called an endocrine gland, that is released into the blood and transported to another organ or tissue, where it performs a specific action. Examples of hormones are insulin, oestrogen, testosterone, and adrenalin.

Hyperglycaemia: An abnormal increase in the amount of sugar in the blood.

Hypertension: High blood pressure.

Hypochondriasis: Mental depression caused by the patient's belief that he or she is suffering from a grave illness, regardless of the accuracy of that belief.

Immune System: A complex system of interlocking substances and tissues that protects the body from disease.

Insomnia: Chronic inability to sleep.

Lesions: Damage to body tissue caused by disease or injury.

Macronutrients: The nurients required in relatively large amounts in the body: protein, carbohydrate, fat, and water.

Micronutrients: The nutrients required in relatively small amounts in the body: vitamins and minerals.

Mineral: An inorganic, fundamental substance found naturally in the soil with specific chemical and structural characteristics.

Osteoporosis: Loss of calcium from the bone that results in reduced bone strength and increased fractures. The bone maintains the same diameter but becomes less dense.

Oxalates: Compounds in some plants that bind to minerals in the body and reduce their absorption.

Ozone: A highly reactive modification of oxygen whereby the two oxygen atoms in oxygen (O_2) are increased to three (O_3).

Pellagra: A disease caused by a deficiency of niacin and characterised by dermatitis, mental disorders, diarrhoea, and weakness.

Phytate: A compound in unleavened whole grains that binds to minerals in the intestines and inhibits their absorption.

Platelets: Cell fragments in the blood that aid in blood clotting,

Rancid: Decomposition of fat characterised by an offensive smell or taste.

Scurvy: A disease caused by a deficiency of vitamin C and characterised by bleeding gums, small haemorrhages under the skin, and weakness.

Tannin: Tannic acid. A yellowish astringent compound found in tea.

Varicose Veins: Enlarged and twisted veins that can occur anywhere in the body, but are most common in the legs.

Vitamin: An organic substance essential to life and required by the body in minute amounts.

Xeropthalmia: A disease caused by a deficiency of vitamin A and characterised by a thickening and inflammation of the outer layers of the eye and impaired eyesight.

Vitamins Checklist –
Needs and Sources

Vitamin A
Daily requirement
    adults   up to 1mg
    children   0.4mg rising to 1mg
Sources
    4oz./110g ox liver   6.8mg
    4oz./110g cooked carrots   2.25mg
    1 halibut liver oil capsule   1.2mg
    4oz./110g cooked spinach   1.15mg

Vitamin B1 (thiamin)
Daily requirement
    adults   1.25mg
    children   0.5mg rising to 1mg
Sources
    1oz./25g cereal + 4fl.oz./
       ½ cup semi-skim milk   0.4mg
    1 large slice of bread   0.15mg
    4oz./110g potato   0.1mg

Vitamin B2 (riboflavin)
Daily requirement
    adults   1.5mg
    children   0.8mg rising to 1.5mg
Sources
    4oz./110g liver   3.5mg

6oz./160g cabbage or Brussels sprouts	1.5mg
1oz./25g cereal + 4fl.oz./½ cup semi-skim milk	0.6mg
1 egg	0.25mg

Vitamin B6 (pyridoxine)

Daily requirement

adults	2mg
children	1.5mg rising to 2mg

Sources

1 banana	480mg
1 orange	90mg
1 egg	50mg

NB Remember that Vitamin B6 is destroyed by heat, light and air.

Vitamin B12

Daily requirement

adults and children	3 micrograms

Sources

6oz./160g meat	2 micrograms
1oz./25g cereal + 4fl.oz./ ½ cup semi-skim milk	1 microgram
8fl.oz./1 cup milk	1 microgram

Folic Acid

Daily requirement

adults and children	400 micrograms

Sources

1 tablespoon brewers yeast	313 micrograms
4oz./110g cooked spinach	165 micrograms
6fl.oz. orange juice	102 micrograms
1oz./25g cereal + 4fl.oz./ ½ cup semi-skim milk	80 micrograms

NB Remember that pregnant women, nursing mothers and women taking an oral contraceptive need extra folic acid.

Niacin
Daily requirement

men	18mg
women	13mg
children	6mg rising to 18mg

Sources

6oz./160g beef	12mg
1oz./25g cereal + 4fl.oz./ ½ cup semi-skim milk	4.6mg
1oz./25g cheese	1.75mg
1 egg	1.65mg

Vitamin C
Daily requirement

adults	30mg–60mg
children	15mg–30mg

Sources

4oz./110g fresh blackcurrants	220mg
1 orange	60mg
4oz./110g Brussels sprouts	40mg

Vitamin D
Daily requirement

adults	10 micrograms
children	7.5 micrograms

Sources

cod liver oil capsule (check dose)	up to 10 micrograms
1oz./25g cereal + 4fl.oz./ ½ cup semi-skim milk	0.6 micrograms

NB Remember that much of the vitamin D requirement is satisfied by exposure to normal amounts of sunlight.

Energy and Minerals Checklist – Needs and Sources

Protein

Daily requirement

men	56 grams
women	44 grams

Sources

6oz./160g turkey	55 grams
8fl.oz./1 cup low fat milk	8 grams
1oz./25g cereal + 4fl.oz./ ½ cup semi-skim milk	6 grams
1 slice wholewheat bread	2.5 grams

Calories

Daily requirement

men	2,000 kcal
women	1,500 kcal

NB People taking strenuous physical exercise add up to 1,000 kcal

Sources

6oz./160g grilled steak	350 kcal
6oz./160g roast chicken without skin	24 0kcal
6oz./160g cod or haddock	120 kcal
6oz./160g chips	420 kcal
medium baked potato	150 kcal
1oz./25g slice of bread	70 kcal
1oz./25g butter	225 kcal

1oz./25g cheddar cheese	115 kcal
½ pint/10fl.oz. semi-skim milk	125 kcal
1 chocolate digestive biscuit	85 kcal
½ pint/10fl.oz. beer (bitter)	100 kcal
5fl.oz. dry white wine	95 kcal

Fibre
Daily requirement

adults and children	30 grams

Sources

1 orange	5.4 grams
1 medium baked potato	5.2 grams
1 slice wholewheat bread	2.7 grams
2 slices wholewheat crispbread	2.6 grams
1oz./25g bran flakes + 4fl.oz./ ½ cup semi-skim milk	2.5 grams

Calcium
Daily requirement

adults	500mg
teenagers and pregnant women	1,200mg

Sources

3oz./80g boiled spinach	500mg
8fl.oz./1 cup milk	300mg
1oz./25g cheese	250mg
1oz./25g cereal + 4fl.oz./ ½ cup semi-skim milk	160mg
1 tablespoon non-fat dried milk	52mg

Copper
Daily requirement

adults and children	2mg

Sources

6oz./160g ox liver	4.75mg
8fl.oz./1 cup whole milk	0.09mg

Iron
Daily requirement
    adults and children   12mg
Sources
    1oz./25g cereal + 4fl.oz./
       ½ cup semi-skim milk   2.1mg

Potassium
Daily requirement
    adults and children   2–3 grams
Sources
    1oz./25g cornflakes + 4fl.oz./
       ½ cup semi-skim milk   200mg
    1oz./25g oatmeal   111mg
    8fl.oz./1 cup whole milk   340mg

Sodium
Daily requirement
    adults and children   1–3 grams
Sources
    1 teaspoon salt   2.3 grams
    1oz./25g cornflakes + 4fl.oz./
       ½ cup semi-skim milk   400mg
    1oz./25g oatmeal   10mg
    7oz./200g baked beans   1 gram

Zinc
Daily requirement
    adults and children   10mg
Sources
    6oz./160g ox liver   7.2mg
    1oz./25g cheese   1.1mg
    8fl.oz./1 cup milk   0.93mg

Index